DEMYSTIFYING HOSPICE

Empowering Patients and Supporting
Caregivers Through the Hospice Experience

Petergay Dunkley-Mullings RN

ISBN: 978-1-948777-47-6

Table of Contents

INTRODUCTION

Goal of the Book

In the pages of this book, you'll find a dual purpose—a guiding light for both patients and caregivers. It's not just a guide but a beacon of wisdom and clarity, helping patients demystify what lies ahead, learn how to navigate their symptoms, and providing caregivers insights into the hospice system, with its wealth of services for patients and caregivers alike.

Through this journey, you will gain a deeper understanding of how to infuse life into each day, even when we can't add more days to life. Both patients and caregivers will learn about managing symptoms during this sacred journey. And caregivers, you will learn how to avoid that all-too-common burnout. Through this cooperative effort, this harmonious dance, patients will discover ultimate comfort in their final stages of life, and caregivers will find fulfillment, knowing they've been a supportive, present pillar for their loved ones.

For patients stepping into the realm of hospice care, this book will shed light on the expectations, procedures, and actions that become your guideposts. For example, should you be caught in the grip of pain, you'll learn the first steps to take. And if those steps don't lead you to the comfort you seek, you'll find guidance on what to do next. This wisdom will teach you when to reach out—be it to your hospice company, your social worker, your chaplain, or even to request an increase in visits from your nursing assistant.

And caregivers, we haven't forgotten you. To help you replenish your energies, the hospice system offers respite services. The patient can be moved to a facility for five days, allowing much-needed rest and rejuvenation. This is available monthly and can be arranged as often as needed.

As we navigate these pages together, know that this book is also a resource for nurses and administrators alike. If your hospice company seeks my guidance as a consultant to educate your staff, this book will be the roadmap for our shared learning journey.

Our primary audience is you, the caregivers—the nurses, doctors, family, and others who support individuals at life's end. We may not always address the patients directly, but the advice you'll find within is all about supporting you in how to discuss hospice services and procedures with your patients. Included are questionnaires to guide your conversations with your patients, providing you with the tools to bring clarity and understanding to their journey.

Expect the Unexpected

Miriam, A New Friend

I started in hospice care at a time when I was *really*, really afraid of death and dying, and I was horrified by even the thought of being in the same room with somebody who's dying.

My first instructor in nursing school saw my fear and thought that I should face it. So, she assigned me to a hospice floor. I remember my first shift vividly. As I stepped off the elevator, I felt death in the air. With trepidation, I walked to the nurse's station and the charge nurse said I would be looking after Miriam [1], a patient with heart disease who had been in hospice for six days. Jane, my mentor nurse that night, was a stern lady who lacked compassion, perhaps because she was looking after three patients and was stretched thin emotionally.

Miriam was at the end of the hall in room five and had a habit of repeatedly pressing her call button. As soon as I arrived, Miriam was paging a nurse—again—so, Jane curtly said, "Follow me." I could tell by her demeanor that she was tired of Miriam's demands. This time, Miriam wanted pain medication, but it was too soon for another dose. Jane said to Miriam, "I can't give you any more pain medication. I've already given it to you, and it's not time for your next dose." Then, much to my horror, Jane took the call button away from Miriam so that she couldn't call the nurse's station anymore.

Back at the nurse's station, I sat there for a few minutes in a quandary. I was not in a position to question Jane's actions, but I felt empathy for Miriam. Finally, I asked, "Do you mind if I go to sit with Miriam?" I'm sure Jane was glad to get rid of me and said sure. So, I went and sat with Miriam. I asked her, "What's really going on? Are you having physical pain or are you just

---

1 All names have been changed to protect the privacy of all people mentioned in this book.

sad because you're in hospice?" Miriam broke down and started telling me her story.

I learned that Miriam was from Cuba, that she migrated here with one daughter and spent all her money on this daughter. She said the daughter got "Americanized," and didn't care about family anymore (that was her interpretation of being Americanized). Miriam lamented that now she was here, all alone, dying. I said, "No, you're not dying." In my naivety, I thought since she looked fine, she was fine. We had a wonderful conversation and bonded right away. I spent the whole night with her.

At the end of my shift, in the wee hours of the morning, I reported to my instructor. I told her I had such a great night and had met a lovely lady who told me her story. My instructor said, "So you see, hospice is not that bad."

The next day, I asked my instructor if I could go back to the same floor and be with Miriam again. She agreed, so I ran upstairs, with a few treats in hand for Miriam, thinking what a blast we'd have that night. I whizzed by the nurse's station and threw open Miriam's door. Her room was empty. Confused, I went back to the nurse's station and asked where Miriam had been moved to. The charge nurse told me that Miriam had died.

Unbeknownst to me, her body was being taken down on the gurney in the elevator as I was racing up to see her. Through my shock and numbness, there was clarity in my mind; I thought putting somebody in a room to fade away and die alone was not right. Everyone needs companionship and tenderness in their final hours. At that moment, I decided to be a hospice nurse and the best hospice nurse possible—one with compassion. I knew I would never treat anybody the way I saw Jane treat Miriam.

When I told my instructor I wanted to do hospice, she asked me why. I said, "Because I met a friend who was hurting on the inside, and I was able to ease her pain." Often, dogs are treated better than Miriam was. I wanted to make sure that I was that nurse who would sit with the next Miriam and be present for her. I would sit, talk, and interact with patients. I would do all the things that I didn't get to do with my new friend, Miriam, who died alone.

So, despite my fear of being around death, straight out of nursing school, my very first job was in hospice, and that's what I've been doing ever since.

My Son

My career in the death care industry has been anchored in love, care, and genuine concern for patients, as well as their families, because I experienced deep pain surrounding the death of my son.

My son had a virus, just a common flu with a fever. Two other children in our neighborhood died two weeks apart with RSV, an upper respiratory infection, so my son may have had that, too. In our tradition, when someone had a high fever, they would be given medication and then wrapped in a blanket. The theory was that the disease would be sweated out. Later, as a nurse, I learned that the correct way to combat a fever is to remove all of the patient's clothes and try to cool them down. Growing up, my mom had treated all six of her kids, including me, with the wrap-and-sweat technique, and none of us had died. I never even questioned this technique as my son was wrapped to sweat out his disease. By the time his seizures started, it was too late. He died as we sat cradling him, waiting for the doctor to come.

He was only three years and seven months old when he died. I remember to this day when I went to identify him for the autopsy. The medical examiner's assistant picked him out of a cold metal tray and dropped him onto an examination table. Yes, literally dropped my precious baby's body; it made a heart-wrenching thud that still echoes in my ears.

Horrified and taken aback, I said to the assistant, "You didn't have to drop him like a piece of meat!"

She callously said, "I'm sorry, but he's already gone."

The death industry can be cold and harsh, but it can also be warm and peaceful. The experience of my son being treated like trash and Miriam being treated without dignity in her final days was incomprehensible to me. I felt a calling to provide patients, as well as their families and friends, with compassion on their final journey. There is no reason that our loved ones should be treated poorly or disrespectfully at the end of life.

The experiences helped me pivot in the direction where I *should* be, not where I *wanted* to go initially.

My First Patient

I went to work for hospice straight out of nursing school, knowing that my experience with Miriam was going to guide me throughout my nursing career. The first time one of my patients died, I called my mother first, not my agency. It hit me so hard, and I needed to hear her voice to collect myself. My father managed a funeral home when I was growing up, so my mother was accustomed to discussing death.

As I cried uncontrollably, I blurted out to my mom, "Oh, my God, my patient just died!" Mom was surprised, too.

"What do you mean the patient *died*?"

I repeated, "Mom, the patient died. She's not breathing!" And I started crying again.

Concerned, Mom asked, "Where are you? I hope you're not in the house with her!"

I said, "No, Mom, I'm standing outside." I felt disconnected from what was happening.

Mom said, "You're just like your father." Still unfamiliar with my newfound position in the death care industry, I realized that my mom was right—I was like my father, and I was going to survive this. It truly was a calling, and I needed to come to terms with the reality of death. I needed to overcome my fear and awkwardness facing it.

My short call with Mom felt like it was two hours, but it was only a few minutes. As reality set in, I thought, *Oh, I need to call my company.*

Most people facing death, whether the patient or family, are lost in the unknown. Facing death is not a common everyday experience for people. They have one chance to do it "right"—and "right" looks different for everyone. There's no do-over. It's one time. Experienced hospice nurses and death doulas can bridge the gap between the patients, who may not have a voice at this stage, and their scared families.

With Mom's comforting words, I collected my wits and reached out to the company. They sent a Registered Nurse (RN) out to do the pronouncement of death because I was a Licensed Practical Nurse (LPN) and not qualified to do so at that time.

From my first brush with the eternal cycle of life and death, my trepidation towards death began to diminish. As time journeyed on, my compassion blossomed, my skills evolved, and I became an empathetic custodian to those on the threshold of passing. With over two thousand death pronouncements under my belt, I stand here today, no longer in the shadow of fear but in the embrace of understanding and acceptance.

Hospice Services

Four Levels of Hospice Care

Understanding the four types of hospice care is crucial for both patients and caregivers because knowledge is power. Being well-informed about the options available gives one the ability to advocate for themselves or their loved one and make decisions that are most aligned with their comfort, dignity, and care needs.

From a patient's perspective, having a thorough understanding of the various types of hospice care can help reduce anxiety and fear. It equips you with an understanding of what to expect in different scenarios, providing a sense of control and autonomy in an often uncertain and vulnerable time. It allows you to be proactive in your care plan, ensuring you receive the right kind of support when you need it most.

For caregivers, knowing the different types of hospice care means being better prepared to provide the necessary support to the patient. It enables you to navigate the care system effectively and facilitates more productive conversations with healthcare providers. It means being equipped to make informed decisions, easing the emotional toll of caregiving, and ultimately helping you ensure the best possible quality of life for your loved one.

Routine Home Care

Hospice care should be like the lighthouse in a storm, a beacon of hope and comfort, steadfast and available to all who seek its light, regardless of where they find themselves in life's journey. A patient's "home" could be a traditional house, a nursing home, or an assisted living facility. Yet, it could also be as unconventional as a car or even a homeless encampment. The call for nationwide hospice services, accessible to all terminally ill patients irrespective of their living conditions, is a fundamental principle we must uphold.

Unfortunately, some hospice agencies fail to extend their services to our homeless brothers and sisters, a practice that should be rectified. No matter the circumstances, every life deserves compassion, dignity, and care.

Routine home care plays an essential role for patients at life's sunset who aren't wrestling with distress or debilitating symptoms. They are known to be at the end of life, yet they are in a place of relative comfort. The goal here isn't so much intervention but monitoring, supporting, and being present. It's like a vigilant shepherd, quietly watching over the flock, ready to step in when needed but respectful of their peace when it's not.

These patients will enjoy the comforting presence of their case manager once or twice a week. Much like an artist studying a canvas, the case manager will carefully review all medications and symptoms, painting a holistic picture of the patient's level of well-being. Being there, watching, and understanding becomes a source of comfort, a bridge between the patient and the best care they deserve.

Respite Care

Respite care is the balm to the weariness of a caregiver's soul. The path of caregiving can be relentless, a never-ending cycle that demands so much of you physically, emotionally, and mentally. It's a role that keeps you on your toes, one that's akin to being on-call every moment of every day. It's no surprise then that exhaustion can settle in, making it imperative to seek respite and restoration.

Hospice steps in like a friend extending a helping hand, offering to transport the patient to a welcoming facility. For five transformative days, the patient receives care away from home. This period is not just about providing necessary care to the patient, but it's also about creating an oasis of calm and rejuvenation for the caregiver.

Imagine it as a restorative retreat—an opportunity to recharge, to indulge in self-care, and to remember who you are outside of the caregiving role. The beauty of this system is its cyclical nature. This respite care can occur every one to two months, availability permitting, ensuring regular intervals of self-renewal for the caregiver.

Think of it as the rhythmic ebb and flow of the sea. Just as the sea withdraws to gather strength before rushing back to the shore with renewed energy, so does the caregiver retreat into the sanctuary of respite care, gathering strength and returning to their role with renewed vigor, empathy, and resilience.

Continuous Care (aka Crisis Care)

When we talk about continuous care, also known as crisis care, we're addressing those patients who are riding the wave of persistent physical symptoms. It might be the relentless tide of nausea, the whirlwind of vomiting, the piercing torrent of uncontrolled pain, the unsettling storm of diarrhea, the heatwave of fever, the unexpected shock of seizures. These battles can't be sufficiently addressed with just a visit or two each week.

So, what does hospice do? It steps up. It leans in. It commits to providing a nurse whose mission is to sit at the patient's bedside, to be a rock, a safe harbor amid their storm. This nurse becomes their confidante, their warrior, and their champion, standing by them for as long as it takes to manage these symptoms.

But here's the thing: if that nurse, after a day or two, is still battling those persistent symptoms despite all the interventions, despite all the tools in their arsenal, we recognize that it's time for a strategic shift. It's time to level up and move to the next stage of care. Because no matter what, the mission remains the same: providing the best care possible for every patient, every single time.

General Inpatient Care

When the river of physical discomfort begins to surge, sometimes a patient finds themselves in need of a deeper level of care: a constant, vigilant presence to help manage their pain and symptoms. This is where General Inpatient Care steps in, like a dependable shelter in a storm.

The patient is gently transitioned from the familiarity of their home to the healing haven of a care facility. This move allows for ongoing, hands-on intervention that caters to their immediate and persistent needs. Like a lovingly woven blanket of care, around-the-clock attention is provided, the rhythm of this constant care echoing in the administering of medications via IVs.

This level of hospice care isn't just about managing the physical journey; it's about providing an enveloping presence, ensuring that every patient feels seen, heard, and comforted even during their trials.

Each of the four levels of hospice care comes with its unique set of participation conditions, rules, and regulations, all put in place by Medicare and Medicaid. These are not just red tape or bureaucratic hoops to jump through. Rather, they are the guidelines that hospice providers are bound to follow, ensuring the provision of care is consistent, comprehensive, and compassionate.

When patients and caregivers have a clear understanding of these hospice care services, it's like having a reliable compass in uncharted territory. It equips them with the knowledge to make informed choices, allowing them to navigate their journey with confidence and autonomy.

This comprehension isn't just a tool, it's a catalyst. It empowers the management of the end-of-life process with grace and dignity, helping to foster a peaceful and respectful experience. By understanding the intricacies of hospice care, we can make sure every person's journey ends not just in comfort, but also with a reaffirmed sense of humanity and self-determination.

Reflection Questions: Hospice Service

1. List three strategies you'd use to help your family cope and stay informed during the hospice journey

   _____

   _____

   _____

2. Which care level feels right for your dear one's current needs?

   _____

   _____

   _____

3. Considering Continuous Care, how might it comfort your loved one, and what steps can you take to ensure they feel supported?

   _____

   _____

   _____

The Hospice Admissions Packet

Imagine setting foot on a new, unexplored land without a map or guide. You might feel lost, uncertain, or even overwhelmed. The Hospice Admissions Packet serves as your trusted guide, your map in this unfamiliar landscape.

When you take the time to dive into the details, to absorb and value this packet, you empower yourself. You replace uncertainty with understanding, fear with familiarity. This packet, complete with its literature and E-Kit, is more than just words and a list of medications. It's a promise. A promise of guidance, support, and knowledge. The packet provides you with vital insights about the journey ahead, insights that can shape your perspective, alleviate anxieties, and equip you to make informed decisions.

It's like finding a torch in the dark, a compass in the unknown. Reading and valuing this packet is an act of self-care, of self-love. It's you saying, "I choose to walk this path with my eyes wide open. I choose to be informed, to be prepared, to be engaged." Because every journey, including the journey of hospice care, is less daunting when we understand the path we're walking.

Literature

Imagine the Patient and Family Care guide as your personal GPS for this journey. While each agency may add its unique flair, the core essence remains the same—a rich compendium of essential insights and guidance that light your path. Yes, it might have as many as 80+ pages, yet it's worth exploring each one of them. Take your time, soak in the wisdom, and truly digest the knowledge it offers.

Within these pages, you may find a space dedicated to your thoughts, questions, and important notes. This is your canvas. Paint it with your curiosity, your concerns, your ideas. And if the canvas isn't enough, claim more space. Use a notebook, and let your thoughts and questions breathe.

In your packet, you may also find a guiding light named "Gone From My Sight, The Dying Experience" by Barbara Carnes. This is not a prophecy but a lantern illuminating the possible twists and turns of the end-of-life journey. It shares common signs and symptoms to help prepare families and caregivers for what might unfold.

Also nestled within your packet is a thoughtful guide for the final two weeks of life. This part of the journey has many names, but for the sake of our journey together, we'll call it "Sacred Journey Care."

Seasoned hospice nurses are skilled in recognizing the subtle signs of transition, be it weeks, days, or mere hours away. When the time draws near, families are encouraged to visit, and the hospice team increases their visits, ensuring daily support.

As the journey nears its end, fear and anxiety may surface, but know that you're not alone. The hospice team's daily presence is a comforting blanket, providing reassurance and space to process the unfolding events.

Also in your pack, you'll discover an Emergency Kit (E-Kit), akin to a guardian angel in a box. This comfort kit holds medications designed to ease common end-of-life symptoms. Comprehensive training accompanies this kit, empowering caregivers with the knowledge to administer these medications confidently.

Each E-Kit is tailored to the patient's needs and is housed in a compact white box or plastic bag. From alleviating pain to soothing agitation, every aspect is covered. For those times when a patient cannot swallow, alternative routes of medication administration are discussed, ensuring comfort and respect are maintained throughout.

Understanding the contents of your hospice packet is like unlocking a chest of knowledge and resources. Take the time to familiarize yourself with each element, embracing the empowerment that comes with knowledge.

A typical E-Kit will include:

Symptom	Typical Medications
Severe Pain	Morphine, Dilaudid
Fever	Tylenol (Acetaminophen)
Nausea	Zofran
Vomiting	Promethazine/Zofran
Shortness of Breath	Morphine
Anxiety / Agitation	Lorazepam
Excessive Oral Secretions	Levsin
Constipation	Bisacodyl
Seizures	Lorazepam

In the realm of hospice care, an around-the-clock support system of nurses is readily available seven days a week. Yet, there will be times when immediate attention is required for the patient's comfort. If a dose or two of the medication doesn't bring the desired relief, that's when you reach out to a hospice nurse.

The essence of the role a family member plays is ensuring the physical and emotional comfort of their loved one. Their duties might involve keeping their loved one clean and comfortable, ensuring they are well-fed and groomed, and overall making certain they are safe. Everything that has been done prior to entering hospice care is expected to continue. As for hospice visits, they are usually short and precise, with the CNA needing just an hour or two to fulfill their responsibilities. Hospice takes on the role of providing all necessities to ensure comfort for the patients, from medications to the hospital bed.

Hospice care is all about empowering family members and care-givers. It's about instilling in them the confidence to care for their loved ones and manage their symptoms effectively. But you are never alone in this. Hospice is always available to answer your queries, guide you through concerning situations, and provide additional help whenever required. We are there for you every step of the way.

A Typical Hospice Timeline

Disclaimer: A prognosis of six months or less is only a quali-fying marker for hospice eligibility. However, a lot of patients in hospice will live for years; some patients even get discharged from hospice if their condition improves.

Stepping into hospice care can be overwhelming, but under-standing the timeline helps you navigate this important pas-sage. Let me take you on a journey from when the diagnosis is pronounced to when hospice care takes the helm.

Envision the starting point of this journey: a place where patients may be living independently, managing their day-to-day tasks alone. Or they may have part-time caregiving assistance, live with a dedicated caregiver, or reside in a care facility, such as an independent living complex, group home, or nursing home.

Consider those living alone, possibly forgoing regular doctors' appointments until an event—maybe a bout of the flu, a stroke—whisks them off to urgent care. Here, they receive the life-altering news that they are living with a terminal illness. These individuals may walk into hospice care unaccompanied.

Then imagine those already in the arms of caregiving—those who, under the watchful eyes of others, discern the presence of a terminal illness early and already have a care structure in place.

Regardless of the onset—whether the diagnosis is fresh or has been a relentless shadow for years—and no matter if they stand alone or are bolstered by a team, once they enter hospice, the system adapts to their needs, providing medical services and extending a supportive hand to their loved ones, who serve as caregivers.

This care may unfold within the familiar walls of the patient's home or within a care facility. In cases where the caregivers are medically trained staff at inpatient facilities, the hospice care transition takes on a unique dynamic.

Now, let's imagine the patient's journey into hospice care.

Hospice Care Timeline:

Month 0: Diagnosis and prognosis of six months or less is given. The individual may start researching hospice care providers, electing hospice care instead of seeking aggressive and curative measures, continuing to live independently, with part-time help, or in a full-time care facility.

Month 1-2: The patient or their loved ones begin to explore hospice care options, possibly exploring respite care to alleviate caregiver burnout and stress.

Month 3-4: The patient and their caregivers adjust to the new routine of hospice care, with regular visits from the hospice team, nurses, social workers, CNAs, and spiritual counselors.

Month 5-6: As the patient nears the end of life, the hospice team increases support, visiting daily to provide comfort, medical attention, and emotional and spiritual support to the patient and their loved ones.

End of Life: The hospice team remains present or available by phone, providing comfort and guidance to the patient and their family during this challenging time.

The Hospice Care Team

Overview

When we step into the world of hospice care, it's akin to walking into an ensemble cast where each member carries a pivotal role. The story that unfolds is unique to each person, a deeply personal narrative of compassion, strength, and grace. Understanding how to navigate this diverse team and harness its collective strength is essential in ensuring this journey is not traversed alone but in partnership with a cadre of individuals dedicated to our care and support.

Imagine you're the director of your life's movie, one that is now pivoting toward a chapter of surrender and transformation. The importance of understanding and navigating your hospice care team lies in the fact that this team forms the core supporting cast. They are the people who will join you in this new terrain, ready to lend their expertise and care in making this journey meaningful, manageable, and as comfortable as possible.

The case manager, visit nurses and CNAs, social workers, bereavement coordinator, chaplain, and doctors—each one is a piece of a puzzle that completes your circle of support. They bring their unique gifts and specialties, creating a comprehensive shield of care. But what's important here is not just knowing what they do. It's about understanding how their energies align with your needs and desires and how you can lead the collective efforts to create an environment that resonates with your comfort, peace, and dignity.

Hospice care is a dance where everyone has a part to play. The tempo and rhythm may change over time, but every role matters and contributes to the harmonious flow of care. Learning to navigate this dance and directing the energies and talents of the team is where your empowerment lies.

Imagine being able to converse with your case manager in a way that you both clearly understand each other's language. You grasp their medical jargon, and they understand your fears, aspirations, and the nuances of your comfort. It's about building relationships with your social workers, who can align resources to your unique needs, and the chaplain who can support your spiritual journey. It's about understanding the visit nurses and CNAs and learning to express your physical needs effectively. It's about harnessing the wisdom of the bereavement coordinator to guide your loved ones as they navigate their emotional journey.

This understanding is not a one-way street. It's a reciprocal process. By understanding your hospice team, you empower them to understand you better. They are then able to provide care tailored to your specific needs and desires. You form a partnership with them in your care, fostering an environment of trust, respect, and mutual understanding.

Recognizing the significance of this understanding helps foster dialogue, enabling you to articulate your fears, preferences, and expectations. It encourages you to ask the tough questions and to expect transparency and empathy. When you understand your team, you are equipped to actively participate in the decisions that affect your life and well-being, which is the very essence of empowerment.

In essence, knowing how to build and navigate your hospice care team ensures that you remain the lead actor in your story, even in this poignant, transformative chapter of your life. The script may seem daunting, the emotions overwhelming, and the process disorienting, but remember, you're not alone. You are surrounded by your team, your supporting cast, who are there to ensure that your voice is heard, your dignity preserved, and your journey is undertaken with respect and love.

It's about creating a symphony where every instrument and note contributes to a beautiful composition. You're the maestro, and your hospice team are your musicians. Understanding how to navigate and work with your team empowers you to orchestrate a hospice experience that respects your journey, values your life, and meets your unique needs.

Once patients enter hospice services, there is an interdisciplinary approach to their care utilizing a team comprised of:

- Doctors who are the patient's primary physician and medical director
- Case Manager (a qualified Registered Nurse)
- Visit Nurses who could either be LPNs or RNs
- Certified Nursing Assistants (CNA)
- Social Workers
- Bereavement Coordinator
- Chaplain

A case manager, always a Registered Nurse ("RN"), oversees the entire case. They are the primary point person for the hospice team and are responsible for the patient's care. The case manager pilots the care plan on the clinician side, is responsible for assigning the social workers, the Visit Nurses, CNAs, social workers bereavement coordinators, and chaplains, and holds regular team meetings to ensure all disciplines are fulfilling their roles.

On the nursing side, the RN (also the case manager), is supported by Visit Nurses and CNAs who go to the home or wherever the patient calls home to provide multiple services. RNs and Visit Nurses provide overall health assessments and symptom management—they do dressing changes, wound care, prescription medication checks, and so on. The CNAs help patients with

Activities of Daily Living (ADLs), such as bathing, dressing, brushing their teeth, fluid and nutritional intake, mobility, and elimination needs. Sometimes, they give gentle massages while checking to make sure that their skin is intact. Physical touch comforts many patients and should only be done with permission.

Patients also have a bereavement coordinator and a non-denominational chaplain for spiritual support. Whatever denomination the patients are from, the chaplain will cater to that spiritual aspect. The chaplain will officiate funerals when the deceased patient didn't have a pastor. The bereavement coordinator supervises the chaplains. The bereavement coordinator is responsible for administrative tasks, such as making sure letters are sent out and following up with the family to see if they need anything. They also coordinate schedules and remind the chaplain to administer a word of prayer and when to be present for the family to talk. In some cases, the bereavement coordinator and chaplain roles are filled by the same individual.

The patient's care team also includes a social worker who will go and sit with the family and review the finances to determine what resources are available to them. Some patients qualify for Medicaid and other benefits. Social workers will know what local resources can be utilized, such as Meals on Wheels, companion sitters (which hospice doesn't provide), and other organizations that can help patients and their families.

In hospice, we take an interdisciplinary approach. So, for example, for any one patient, we have a team that takes care of this patient. We have a medical doctor and a nurse practitioner. We have our own case managers or registered nurses who manage the caseload for our patients who will be assigned to an individual patient. And he or she will manage the entire process. Working with this registered nurse, we do have a social worker as well as a chaplain, and a certified nursing assistant.

The doctors review the patient's care plan every two weeks. The registered nurse makes visits at least once a week. That increases when patients are transitioning towards the end of life; when they have two or three weeks left, nurses and social workers do daily visits. The certified nursing assistant also visits anywhere from three to five days a week, where he or she will go to the homes and provide basic comfort care like bathing, dressing, and feeding—anything outside of the pharmacological intervention. We also have a 24-hour line where the patients or their families can call in with questions and receive support. There's a whole team taking care of each patient in hospice.

In order to be a hospice case manager, the individual must be a registered nurse. As for certification, I encourage nurses who are interested in hospice care to get a hospice and palliative care certification. The palliative aspect is very important because it really helps nurses learn about palliative medicine and palliative care in terms of caring for the patients, as well as the families.

Team Meetings – Open to All

All hospice services hold team meetings at least every two weeks to ensure that all service disciplines work smoothly together for the patient's benefit. These team meetings are referred to as Interdisciplinary Team (IDT) meetings or Interdisciplinary Group (IDG) meetings. Holding these meetings is one of the conditions of participation in the Medicare / Medicaid program. All disciplines, including the doctor, the case manager / RN, all other nurses involved except the CNA who provides personal care, all chaplains, and bereavement coordinators attend the meetings.

These meetings are open to CNAs, and they often attend to stay abreast of treatment plans for their patients. Also, the meetings are open to caregivers, although that is not widely known. To protect the privacy of patients, when caregivers choose to attend the meetings, they are called in when we discuss their loved ones. It is a wonderful opportunity for caregivers to hear from the entire care team, ask questions, and get a full picture of the patient's condition. I encourage people to utilize this option fully.

Doctors

In the realm of hospice care, doctors play a vital role in ensuring compassionate support for patients and their families. These healthcare professionals bring their expertise, knowledge, and heartfelt commitment to providing comfort and dignity during the final stages of life. Let's delve into the essential role doctors play within the hospice care journey.

Expert Medical Care

Doctors in hospice care bring a wealth of medical knowledge and experience to the table. They are responsible for evaluating patients' medical conditions, monitoring symptoms, and collaborating with the case manager, who will develop personalized care plans. Doctors take a holistic approach to patient care, from managing pain and providing relief from distressing symptoms to addressing emotional and spiritual needs. They work closely with the interdisciplinary hospice team to create comprehensive treatment plans that prioritize the patient's comfort and well-being.

Communication and Coordination

Effective communication and coordination are essential aspects of a doctor's role in hospice care. Doctors collaborate with patients, families, and the interdisciplinary team to ensure everyone is informed and aligned with the care plan. They provide clear explanations about the patient's condition, treatment options, and the goals of hospice care. Additionally, doctors advocate for patients, ensuring their wishes and preferences are respected and integrated into the care process.

Medication Management

Medication management is critical to hospice care, and doctors play a key role in overseeing this aspect. They prescribe medications to alleviate pain, manage symptoms, and improve the patient's overall quality of life. Doctors carefully monitor the effectiveness of medications, adjusting dosages or changing prescriptions as needed. They work closely with case managers and pharmacists to ensure that medications are readily available and delivered in a timely manner.

Support for Caregivers

Doctors in hospice care also extend their support to caregivers who play a significant role in providing care and comfort to patients. They offer guidance and education to caregivers, empowering them with the knowledge and skills necessary to effectively manage the patient's care at home. Doctors understand the challenges and emotional toll that caregiving can bring, and they provide reassurance, empathy, and encouragement to caregivers, helping them navigate the journey with confidence.

Case Managers (RN)

The case manager for each patient is a registered nurse. They direct and oversee the patient's care throughout their transition journey. The case manager formulates the care plan based on the patient's health status and goals and will continually assess the situation and adjust the plan as needed throughout the journey. They will recommend resources as needed and will advocate on the patient's behalf.

The case manager employs skills beyond their RN medical training. They approach hospice care wholistically with the patient's physical, mental, emotional, and spiritual well-being in mind. Case managers act as an anchor for the team and directs each team member in their role to ensure the patient is best served.

The care plan details the frequency of visits for each of the team members. For example, a patient may initially need two visits a week from the CNA, once-a-month visits from the social worker, alternating with once-a-month visits from the chaplain. Visits will sometimes decrease (if the patient temporarily improves), but more often, the visits increase as the patient's health declines.

Depending on the patient's health, the case manager will typically visit weekly or biweekly. At the end of life, when the patient enters Sacred Journey Care, the RN will visit every day, seven days a week. Most case managers work Monday through Friday, so on weekends, hospice will send another on-call RN who is knowledgeable about the case and follows the case manager's directives.

Case manager visits usually start with an assessment of the patient's symptoms. They determine if the patient is having any pain, has diarrhea, is running a fever, has seizures, and so on. Usually, the patient is suffering from one or more symptoms, so the nurse will discuss each one.

For instance, if the patient reports being in pain, the nurse will ask questions to understand the level and frequency of the pain, and then compare it to medications taken. The case manager relays this information to the doctor and can advocate for a prescription adjustment. When a patient has been taking morphine as prescribed but is still in pain and the RN reports that to the doctor, the doctor may decide to increase the dosage and/or frequency of the medication.

A case manager constantly reviews the situation and looks for opportunities to better serve the patient and control their discomfort. When an RN walks into a situation and notices that the patient is restless and anxious, even knowing that the patient may be in denial or doesn't understand what is happening to them (particularly in cases involving dementia), the case manager will review the medications to see what's prescribed for restlessness and anxiety and then make the recommendation for appropriate prescription medications.

Case managers know that in every home, different family dynamics impact the patient. Beyond their skills as RNs, the case managers seek to understand the patient's living situation and will reach out to the social worker when it is likely patients could benefit from a social worker's intervention. For instance, if there is too much stimulation from the family (too many visits, too much noise, etc.), or other potentially upsetting concerns, such as tense relationships, or the patient is being ignored, the social worker can intervene and work towards resolving such issues.

When a case manager knows that a patient has certain religious beliefs, prays regularly, or is having spiritual discontent or anguish, they will reach out to the chaplain and request they visit the patient.

In addition to assessing the patient's well-being weekly, case managers also continually assess the need for community resources. Technically, this is the social worker's role, but case managers' frequent interaction with the patient reveals needs, and they will liaise with the social worker to be sure needs are being met. For instance, a case manager might be aware that a patient has little food in the pantry and know that their finances are strained, so they will alert the social worker to the need rather than simply rely on the social worker to identify the need. Resources for clothing and other household items are also available.

Case managers are more likely to interact with the patient's caregiver and will know if that individual is available 24/7, or is juggling their time with other obligations. When a caregiver has a job, other family obligations, or other outside responsibilities, hospice can suggest companion resources. For our veteran patients, we can refer veteran organizations. It is common for people who are dying to enjoy the companionship of others. It is a time of reflection, and patients often want to share their memories.

Advocacy is a key function of case managers, particularly for high-risk or vulnerable patients. If a case manager walked into a situation where they suspected the patient had been left alone, abused, or neglected, they will intervene to ensure the patient is in a safe environment. During each visit, case managers look out for any sign of abusive behavior and will advocate for the patient and utilize the hospice team to make sure the patient is being treated with dignity and respect.

Developing the Patient's Care Plan

Think about your care plan as your personal script in this transformative stage of life, a script written in your own words and built around your deepest desires and comfort. In essence, it is the embodiment of your voice, your wishes, and your unique path. It is your declaration of how you wish to be supported, cared for, and comforted in your final season of life.

The care plan's development, steered by your RN case manager, forms a crucial dialogue between you and your hospice team. It brings your narrative to the fore and weaves it into the very fabric of your care. It's not just about medical procedures and timelines; it's about your hopes, fears, and the essence of your comfort. It captures your vision of dignity, peace, and respect.

This care plan stands as your guide, informing every decision, every intervention, and every act of compassion that your hospice team brings forth. It encapsulates the holistic nature of hospice care, resonating beyond the physical to emotional, spiritual, and social realms. It helps your hospice team align their expertise with your desires to create a harmonious symphony of care that honors, comforts, and accompanies you with grace in this profound journey.

Developing the patient's care plan isn't just a procedural step. It's an act of empowerment, an act of love. It's the manifestation of your voice in a time when it's most critical. It's about ensuring that this chapter of life echoes with your strength, your choice, and your dignity.

There are no right or wrong answers; these are personal choices based on each patient's personality, situation, and disease. For instance, if a patient normally experiences pain on a 6-to-8 scale, they may choose to have medication that completely resolves the pain, even if it makes them drowsy. Another patient may choose to live with pain at a 2-to-4 level if it means they are more alert and can interact with their family.

Another important question is what they want done, if anything, if their heart stops. Some people choose to be resuscitated and brought back to life using CPR, intubation, or other invasive means. Others sign a "do not resuscitate order," choosing to transition naturally.

Patients must also indicate how they want to be cared for if their symptoms get to a point where it's difficult to manage them at home. They have the option of continuous home care provided by a nurse, or they can go to the hospital. In my experience, I find that few people want to die in a hospital.

A patient's hospice packet will contain a full list of questions used to develop the care plan. I encourage the patient, and family members or caregivers as appropriate, to carefully consider each question. It is important to remember that the patient's wishes are most important.

When developing the plan, most RNs will spend time reviewing the entire care packet with the patient and family/caregivers and provide example scenarios. I have found that the people who ask the 'what if' questions are best prepared because they take the time to think about various situations.

When patients and families/caregivers receive this training up-front, it usually results in better outcomes and less stress for all involved. There are fewer 'panic' calls, but always know that is what hospice is for—to provide support in emergent and crisis situations. Never hesitate to call your service with questions or concerns.

We have patients who live in nursing homes, and even the trained staff are susceptible to panic, wondering, "Is my patient dying right now?" A hospice nurse is trained to do a quick triage assessment based on six key questions. In an emergency, it is helpful for caregivers to conduct this assessment to accurately report what is happening to the hospice team.

Is the patient in pain? If yes, how severe? (For non-verbal patients, look for non-verbal symptoms of pain—moaning, wincing, grunting or screaming, clenched bodies.)

Is the patient short of breath?
Does the patient have a fever?

Is the patient having seizures?

Does the patient have diarrhea?

Is the patient vomiting?

When the answer is "no" to all these questions, this is an unexpected outcome. I will reach out to the family members, and I will let them know what's going on. And I'm on my way to do an assessment.

Advocating for Patients

Pay attention to the whole person.

Be present as a compassionate caregiver and advocate.

Be a clinician in your head, but let the patient feel your heart.

Listen to what's being said in the background and what's not being said.

Observe how patients are being treated by their caregivers, whether it be paid caregivers or family members.

Notice the interactions between the patients and their family members.

Sometimes, patients are uncomfortable at home and can't speak out for fear of repercussions. When nurses see patients go silent or withdraw when a particular person walks into the room, perhaps their facial expressions change, or they turn away, looking saddened or frightened, the nurse should talk one-on-one in private with the patient.

Ask the patient to explain their emotions, especially concerning ones.

If a patient says, "Maybe when you come tomorrow, I won't be here," or "I just don't want to be here anymore," ask them exactly what they mean. Tell them you are trying to understand their feelings so you can help them. When patients have the opportunity to elaborate on what they're going through it shows them we care and it allows them to provide the information needed to make a decision and advocate for them.

Don't rush. Time is precious for patients, and even if you don't say, "I have to go soon," they can feel your haste.

Don't judge. Provide a safe space for patients to talk about what they're going through.

Best Practices for Case Managers

What do you wish case managers knew that most don't? What's really critical?

Great case managers in hospice care are akin to dedicated architects of hope and bridges of compassion. They hold a sacred responsibility of meticulously weaving a blanket of care around their patients and their families, a blanket that comforts, supports, and honors their unique needs and desires in this deeply personal journey. Let's dive into the elements that characterize exceptional case managers in the world of hospice care.

First and foremost, exceptional case managers lean into empathy. They make it their mission to understand, not merely to respond. They see each patient not as a collection of symptoms but as a unique individual with their own stories, fears, hopes, and dreams. They embrace their role as compassionate listeners, allowing their patients to express their emotions, needs, and wishes openly.

The heart of an exceptional case manager's practice is rooted in advocacy. They become the voice of their patients, ensuring their needs are addressed, their comfort is prioritized, and their wishes are respected. They navigate the complex healthcare system, advocating for resources, services, and decisions that honor the patient's care plan and enhance their quality of life.

Being proactive and anticipatory is a hallmark of exceptional case management. Good case managers understand the ever-evolving nature of end-of-life care and stay steps ahead, anticipating possible challenges, complications, and transitions. They work hand-in-hand with the entire hospice care team to ensure a seamless, coordinated response to the changing needs of their patients.

In the world of hospice care, where the physical, emotional, and spiritual realms intertwine, great case managers adopt a holistic approach. They recognize that care goes beyond the physical symptoms, encompassing the emotional well-being and spiritual peace of their patients. They ensure their care plan addresses these multi-faceted needs, providing a comprehensive, integrated approach to comfort and support.

Excellent case managers are also the orchestrators of communication. They are the nexus connecting patients, families, and the hospice care team, fostering open, transparent, and compassionate dialogues. They understand that clear and timely communication eases anxieties, enhances trust, and promotes a sense of unity and shared purpose.

Finally, an exceptional case manager never forgets the power of presence. They understand that sometimes, the most profound care they can provide is their presence, their attentive silence that conveys understanding, compassion, and shared humanity. They realize that their presence can become a beacon of comfort and connection in times of uncertainty and fear.

In essence, the best practices for case managers in hospice care are framed not only by their professional expertise but also by their deep, heartfelt commitment to compassionate, patient-centered care. It's about more than just managing care; it's about honoring the dignity, voice, and individuality of each patient, ensuring that their final journey unfolds in a space of respect, comfort, and unconditional support.

In a world as delicate as hospice care, the ideal scenario is one where every player on the team operates at their peak, bringing both technical skills and emotional acumen to the field. Unfortunately, this isn't always the reality. Let's explore this by focusing on one particular role: the Visit Nurse, which, when mishandled, can fall into the category of what is known, quite unfortunately, as a "visit nurse."

These individuals tend to be focused on their task lists, clock-watching, and completing their responsibilities as swiftly as possible. The fast pace at which they operate could make their visit seem more like a social call at the expense of thorough assessment and care work. The haste and lack of immersion can compromise the quality of care provided.

Now, let's delve into the roles. Visit Nurses typically offer a supportive role to the case managers, taking on patient interface tasks similar to case managers but without the direct responsibility for individual patients or hospice teams. They are, in essence, the supporting pillars to the case managers, rotating among a larger number of patients.

But herein lies the challenge. These nurses often have a larger pool of patients to care for, which, combined with the inherent time pressures, could inadvertently cultivate a distant and abrupt manner. Such a demeanor could shroud the patient with feelings of discomfort and lack of personal care. This rushed and impersonal approach could make patients feel more like a task to be checked off a list rather than valued individuals whose comfort and well-being are paramount.

I remember working with a nurse who fit the "visit nurse" persona. Despite being aware of this perception, she displayed an apathy toward improving her manner, choosing to stay disconnected and uncompassionate. Her lack of diligence was not only evident in her interaction with patients, but also in her clinical assessments, and this, my dear reader, can be detrimental.

In hospice care, every detail matters. Neglecting to assess something as critical as a wound could escalate the patient's discomfort and possibly compromise their health. When such oversights occur, it falls on the case manager to intervene, retrain, and possibly reprimand the underperforming team member.

The role of a hospice case manager goes beyond ticking boxes on a checklist. It's about empathy, attention to detail, and a deep commitment to patient comfort. It's about communication skills that can liaise effectively with families and training and monitoring skills that ensure the entire team is at its best.

As families navigate through this journey of hospice care, it is crucial to remember that you are not powerless. When you encounter a "visit nurse," someone whose bedside manners may be lacking and who seems more interested in ticking off boxes than being present for the care of your loved one, there are actions that you can, and should, take.

First and foremost, it is essential to remind yourself of the rights your loved one has. They deserve to be treated with respect, dignity, and compassion. Care isn't merely about providing the necessary medications or changing bed linens; it's about the holistic treatment of the patient, considering their emotional, mental, and physical needs. When this expectation isn't met, it is within your rights to seek the care your loved one deserves.

Engage in open conversations with the case manager about your observations and concerns. A well-structured hospice team is built on a foundation of transparency, with case managers playing a crucial role in addressing these concerns. They are equipped to intervene, retrain, and sometimes reprimand team members who may not be fulfilling their roles appropriately.

Additionally, it is essential to communicate directly with the hospice management. They are responsible for ensuring that the team members provide high-quality care and service to all patients. Providing them with the feedback they need to take corrective action is a step in the right direction to improving the overall quality of care.

Furthermore, finding a community or group of individuals who are or have been in similar situations may be helpful. The knowledge and support you can gain from shared experiences can be empowering. Remember, your voice matters, and the changes you instigate could improve the hospice experience for not only your loved one but others as well.

Best Practices for Visit Nurses

Stepping into the sacred sphere of hospice care calls for a deeper dive into humanity. No manual holds all the answers, and there isn't a one-size-fits-all method to caring. Indeed, standards are there and serve as a framework, a compass guiding our work. Still, every home opens up a unique world, with unique needs, and Visit Nurses, must adjust their sails accordingly.

Beginning every visit, one must delve into a comprehensive exploration of the patient - their health, their environment, the pulse of their caregivers, and the dynamics of their familial ties. Every detail paints a picture of their current reality that drives the course of care.

Medications, like subtle brush strokes, often make a significant difference. A Visit Nurse must always inspect the patient's prescriptions to ensure adherence and identify any need for refills.

When we talk about the assessment, it goes beyond a check-and-check routine. It's a pathway to understanding, guiding the case manager in assigning roles, requesting equipment, and shaping the care experience. Detailed and painstakingly thorough, these assessments are not merely boxes to be ticked. They're narratives of our patients' lives.

Yet, we must remember it is not just about being thorough. It's about authenticity. A copy-paste approach can never replace genuine, personalized notes that reflect the true state of each patient. It's not just about efficiency; it's about accuracy and integrity in reporting.

But here's the truth: as Visit Nurses, we might not always get a chance to build deep connections with all our patients. This reality makes it all the more crucial for us to truly see our patients, to pay attention to the subtle details noted by other nurses, to validate them, and to add our own observations.

An assessment isn't just a clinical evaluation. It's a golden opportunity to extend our hearts, empathy, and understanding to our patients. It's a chance to be fully present, to be a light in the lives of those we care for.

Let's reflect on three essential pillars of exceptional nursing care:

1. **Compassion:** As we step into this role, we carry the profound responsibility of caring for another human being. This responsibility demands a heart that feels, empathizes, and extends kindness.

2. **Accountability:** Each action we take, each note we write, and each word we say bears weight. It's about owning our role and fulfilling it with sincerity and professionalism.

3. **Self-care and resilience:** The journey isn't always easy. Sometimes, the light dims, and burnout lurks around the corner. In those moments, remember, it's okay to seek help, to recharge, and to ensure we can continue to serve from a place of wellness.

4. **The path of a Visit Nurse** is filled with opportunities to make a real difference, touch lives, and bring profound com-

fort and care. It's about the doing and the being—the tasks and the humanity—interwoven into a tapestry of compassionate care.

Social Workers

As bearers of an often-misunderstood role, Social Workers carry an arsenal of resources as diverse and multi-faceted as a Swiss Army knife. Each tool they wield serves a unique purpose, tailored to every patient's specific needs. The beauty of their work lies in their capacity to pivot seamlessly, to adapt their approach, to align their expertise with the evolving needs of their patients and families.

The strength of their role is backed by a robust academic foundation, typically a master's degree, which equips them with a deep understanding of the psychosocial dynamics of illness, grief, and loss. But it's more than education that guides them. It's empathy, understanding, and a fierce commitment to humanity.

In the intricate dance of hospice care, the social worker is the choreographer, arranging the elements of care, support, and community resources into a harmonious flow. They are the orchestrators of a connection, ensuring that the necessary resources are not just available, but accessible and well-understood.

At the heart of it all, the hospice social worker serves as a beacon of light, cutting through the fog of uncertainty with expertise, compassion, and commitment. They stand tall in the face of life's most challenging transitions, their hearts echoing the unwavering promise: "You are not alone. We are here with you, for you.

Funeral Arrangement Guidance

When it comes to making final arrangements—a process that's fraught with deep emotions and crucial decisions—the social worker's role is invaluable.

Imagine a lantern in the darkest night, illuminating the path ahead. That's the social worker. They have a vast knowledge of local funeral homes and crematoriums, guiding patients and caregivers through the labyrinth of choices. Each option is an intimate reflection of the patient's journey, their religious beliefs, financial circumstances, and personal preferences.

Decisions on such a sensitive matter are never easy. They are the mirrors that reflect the patient's life, their essence, and their legacy. So, the social worker walks alongside them, delicately weaving a tapestry of understanding, respect, and empathy.

They listen intently, asking questions designed to unveil the patient's innermost wishes. These could involve choosing an officiant, or it could be a question of whether they'd prefer the comforting presence of the hospice chaplain at their final rites.

In the face of financial hardship, the social worker's role takes on another dimension. Like a shield, they protect their patient's dignity, searching for solutions such as indigent burial arrangements. The goal here is not to add more stress to an already trying time but to help lighten the burden, to ensure that every individual, irrespective of their financial situation, is given the respect and dignity they deserve in their final journey.

Medicare / Medicaid Guidance

Navigating the intricate labyrinth of healthcare benefits, especially Medicare and Medicaid, can feel like being caught in a swirling, unending storm. The terminology can be confusing, the regulations are overwhelming, and the fear of missing out on crucial assistance is very real. In this storm, a hospice social worker becomes a shining light amidst the darkness.

Social workers are well-versed in the language of healthcare assistance. They understand the ebb and flow of these systems and can wield their knowledge like a compass, pointing their patients toward the path that best suits their needs.

If a patient doesn't already have Medicare or Medicaid, it's not a dead-end, not a wall that they have to scale on their own. Armed with a robust list of resources, the social worker steps up and guides the patient along the process.

It's more than just guidance. Social workers lean in, shoulder-to-shoulder, with their patients. They help to fill out the often-complicated applications, making sure that every T is crossed and every I is dotted. But their role doesn't end with the submission of paperwork.

They vigilantly monitor the progress, overseeing the process like a shepherd watching over their flock. The goal is to ensure that the patient receives the assistance they so rightly deserve in a timely manner.

Medicare and Medicaid are more than just healthcare plans; they are lifelines for many individuals in hospice care.

Food and Utility Resources

In the dimly lit corridors of financial strain, where breadwinners become patients and households teeter on the precipice of want, a beacon of hope emerges. The social worker, attuned to the silent cries of despair, extends a helping hand, gently guiding those under their care through a maze of resources, ensuring their basic needs are met.

This dance of survival is performed with grace by the social worker. They provide a roadmap, a comprehensive list of aid options, illuminating the path to resources like food stamps and food banks. It's not merely about survival but also about dignity. They act as an advocate for families who, amid the turmoil of a life-limiting illness, find themselves unable to carry the financial burden alone.

The social worker's role extends far beyond merely providing a list. They collaborate, stepping into the fray to negotiate, be it with utility companies or other organizations. Their words, whether spoken over the phone or written in earnest letters, serve as shields against the cold wind of deprivation. They advocate for the continuity of essential services, such as ensuring that lights stay on for patients reliant on oxygen and other such necessities.

They bridge the gap between need and fulfillment, sometimes through services like Meals on Wheels, ensuring that nourishment reaches the doors of those who need it most. Their actions become the lifeline for patients and their families, turning the tides of despair into a river of hope.

The work of social workers is more than a profession; it's a mission.

Caregiver Support

Not all heroes are adept at asking for help. Some caregivers, with hearts ablaze with love and devotion, press on, neglecting their own needs, and losing themselves in the labyrinth of care. Here is where the social worker steps in: the coalescence of empathy and action. They recognize the silent pleas for respite in the weary smiles and heavy eyes, and they answer this call.

They act, not just as observers, but as advocates. Communicating with the case manager, they instigate the provision of respite care, offering a lifeline to the struggling caregivers. The proposal isn't just to find someone to momentarily take over but to provide an environment where patients receive comprehensive care, off-site, transportation included.

The magic of respite care is in its reciprocity. As the patient continues to be cared for safely, the caregiver is given the space to breathe, sleep, and refill their own strength. It's a pause, a precious interval where the caregiver can rejuvenate, gather their forces, and return to their role with renewed vigor.

Social workers, in their myriad roles, foster this culture of mutual care. They ensure that in the compassionate dance of caregiving, no one, not the patient or the caregiver, is left to shoulder their burdens alone. They remind us that even in the throes of struggle, self nourishment is paramount. And in doing so, they weave a fabric of support, both seen and unseen, nurturing the caregivers who nurture us all.

Monitor for Abuse and Neglect

Social workers are often the first to notice any signs of neglect or abuse, making them the lifeline for those whose voices are drowned in vulnerability. Like any other team member in the hospice setting, social workers are duty-bound to report any hint of abuse or neglect, but their role doesn't stop there.

Carrying the baton, social workers often step up to lead the process, reporting the unfortunate incidents to the relevant authorities and vigilantly monitoring the situation. Their mission is protecting and safeguarding their patients, and they are unafraid to take these issues to court if necessary.

When they stand in court, they are not just representatives of the hospice care team; they are the voice of their patients. Their training and expertise in psychosocial dynamics equip them uniquely to navigate these waters. They bring an understanding that goes beyond clinical backgrounds, touching the emotional and psychological facets of the situation.

In this vast spectrum of care, social workers play an invaluable role. They are the guardians at the gates, ensuring that the sanctity of hospice care is upheld and every patient is treated with the dignity, respect, and love they deserve. Their work reminds us that in the heart of service, vigilance and advocacy are as important as tenderness and empathy.

Organizing Companionship

Loneliness can often be a quiet companion, stealthily creeping into the hearts of those who have no family or those who feel particularly alone. Amid the medical necessities and logistical considerations, one aspect of care frequently gets overlooked—the power of companionship, the magic of connection. This, dear ones, is where the social worker steps in, acting as the architect of companionship, bringing light to the shadows of loneliness.

Companionship is more than just filling silence or space. It's about building bridges, creating heart-to-heart connections, and letting our patients know that while their journey may be individual, they are not alone. It's about sharing stories, laughter, tears, and memories. It's about being a comforting presence, a warm hand to hold, an understanding smile, and a listener to their fears, dreams, regrets, and joys. Companionship is, in essence, a reminder of our shared humanity, our intertwined destinies.

Social workers play a vital role in recognizing the need for this life-affirming connection. They seek out volunteer companions who can bring a burst of sunshine to our patients' lives, to make them feel seen, heard, and valued. These hospice volunteers become friends, confidantes, and bearers of shared experiences. They breathe life into rooms, stir up reminiscences, and spark joy in moments that can otherwise feel burdened by solitude.

Let's never underestimate the extraordinary impact of companionship. It can transform a sterile, clinical environment into a cozy sanctuary filled with heartbeats and warmth. It's an essential element of care that wraps around the medicinal and the procedural, reaching directly into the heart of our patients, providing comfort, igniting hope, and reminding them of the beautiful tapestry of human connection in which they are woven. Social workers, as the weavers of these connections, enrich the hospice journey, proving that love and companionship can indeed illuminate even the most challenging paths.

Best Practices for Social Workers

Social workers serve as trusted allies, bearing witness to the diverse tapestry of patients' experiences—their triumphs and challenges, their aspirations and fears, their financial, relationship, and household realities.

Nonetheless, we must remember social workers are human, too. Their hearts, though large and steadfast, are not immune to the complexity of emotions and experiences they encounter. It's easy for personal beliefs, experiences, and judgments to slip into their professional role. Yet, they must stand guard against such intrusions. Every person's journey is unique, and every relationship is a universe unto itself.

One poignant instance comes to mind. A patient's spouse was suspected of infidelity, and the case was handled by a social worker whose own life had been scarred by a similar transgression. Her personal pain clouded her professional lens, leading to unwarranted assumptions and misunderstandings. Let this be a reminder to us all that our personal histories must never shadow the illumination we bring to our patients' lives.

Yet, in my years of experience, such instances are rare. Social workers, in general, are a dedicated, caring lot, who rise to their call of service with an unwavering commitment to their patients.

However, even the most dedicated caregivers require time to rest, rejuvenate, and heal. The intense journey of accompanying someone through their final days, of witnessing life ebb away, can be emotionally draining. Burnout, stress, and overwhelming emotions aren't just possibilities but eventualities if not addressed proactively.

This is where the power of self-care kicks in. It's more than just a buzzword; it's a lifeline. Be it indulging in soothing massages or uplifting mani-pedis, immersing in the tranquility of a candle-lit bath, disconnecting from the digital world, or soaking in the restorative power of sleep and exercise, social workers must allow themselves to take a breather.

And let's remember, there's no shame in asking for help. If a social worker feels the weight of personal bias or burnout creeping in, it's crucial that they communicate their concerns. Declining a case when they cannot serve at their best isn't a sign of weakness but a testament to their commitment to their patients. Their own well-being is not a luxury but a necessity, not just for themselves but for the compassionate care they provide. Self-care is not an act of selfishness but a radical act of self-love that echoes through the corridors of hospice care.

Challenges Face by Social Workers

In the orchestra of healthcare, social workers often find themselves as the unsung heroes—pivotal to the harmony yet sometimes underappreciated. They navigate a world punctuated by pain, hope, and vulnerability, all while wearing a cloak of stoicism. Theirs is a story not often told; their worth not always recognized, especially when placed beside the towering stature of doctors and nurses. This perception often lurks in the public eye, and sometimes, sadly, even within the hospice team itself.

These spirited advocates of compassion are frequently blessed with razor-sharp perceptiveness. In interdisciplinary team meetings, their insightful feedback often adds a humanizing layer to medical science's cold, hard facts. Yet, they may occasionally be perceived as stepping outside their bounds, particularly when offering recommendations concerning patients' physical pain and medication.

Imagine a social worker visiting a patient who is ceaselessly screaming in pain. Their empathetic heart and seasoned wisdom might nudge them to suggest an adjustment to the pain medication. But this might not sit well with some nurses, who could misconstrue this as an undermining of their competency. However, the empathetic lens of social workers can offer valuable insights to enrich patient care, and they need to continue to voice their observations, even when faced with resistance.

This brings us to a fundamental truth: the patient's well-being should always be the shared goal of the hospice team. A concert of different perspectives and expertise, orchestrated in harmony, can offer the best possible care. This requires all players to embrace humility and foster a spirit of collaborative cooperation.

Due to their intimate caregiving roles, nursing assistants often form close relationships with patients. This trust-filled connection allows them to bear witness to patients' stories, their hopes and regrets, their pains and pleasures. Yet, social workers, while being privy to these emotional landscapes, must adhere to the medical directives of doctors and nurses, maintaining a careful balance.

A scenario might illustrate this: if a patient is at risk of an aneurysm, the medical staff may instruct the CNAs not to let the patient sit up or be moved to a wheelchair. The CNAs must comply, even if the rationale behind these directives remains a mystery to them. This is because there's a potential risk of the CNAs or social workers unintentionally causing undue fear in the patient if they discuss the medical risk. Thus, social workers tread this tightrope of empathy and adherence, always in pursuit of their core purpose: patient well-being.

Bereavement Coordinators

Bereavement Coordinators form the very heartbeat of hospice care. In their role, they are often seen as tender souls carrying the mantle of hope, perseverance, and kindness. Much like the silent yet relentless beat of a drum, they set the rhythm for the healing process, continuously offering their unwavering support. These individuals step into the intimate world of loss, offering comfort and understanding in the most challenging of times, but let's not minimize their role to mere consolation. No, my friends, they are much, much more.

Bereavement Coordinators perform a dance of resilience and recovery. When the world seems to have crumbled into a thousand pieces, they are there, holding the space, acknowledging the pain, and yet never letting go of the thread of hope. They aid in rebuilding, not just emotional resilience, but also lives that have been dramatically altered.

From the first days of loss through the following months, the bereavement coordinator operates much like an artist. They mold an environment of empathy, understanding, and resilience, a sanctuary where grief can be acknowledged, understood, and honored. They are the empathetic ear, the comforting voice, and, more than anything, the sturdy pillar of support that individuals can lean on. They provide counsel, not just to the immediate family, but also to friends, and at times, to the entire community.

But here's the crux: the Bereavement Coordinator's role is not a one-size-fits-all endeavor. They tailor their support to the unique needs of each individual. For some, they guide them through the rituals of remembering, helping them find solace in the legacy left behind. For others, they offer tools to rebuild their lives, gently encouraging them to rediscover their identity separate from their loss.

Their role extends beyond the immediate aftermath of loss. Bereavement Coordinators often walk alongside individuals throughout the first year after the passing of a loved one. This period is marked by a myriad of firsts: first birthday without their loved one, first holiday, first anniversary. These milestones can stir up a fresh wave of grief, and bereavement coordinators are there, steady and supportive, helping individuals weather these challenging moments.

In essence, the Bereavement Coordinator is an anchor in the tumultuous sea of grief. They serve as an enduring symbol of resilience and hope, fostering an environment where individuals are empowered to grieve openly and honestly while also gradually moving forward. It's about honoring the past, living in the present, and building towards the future. This, my dear friends, is the role of a Bereavement Coordinator: a catalyst of healing and a beacon of hope amid the darkest hours.

Chaplains

In the universe of hospice care, chaplains represent an essential constellation of hope, faith, and reconciliation. They illuminate a path where life and loss intersect, offering solace to those in their most profound moments of vulnerability.

Chaplains, like harmonious symphonies, provide soothing notes during the cacophony of grief and uncertainty. They tune in to the spiritual needs of each individual, becoming a sanctuary of comfort and a source of spiritual nourishment. Their primary mission is to be present, bringing a serene assurance that no one is alone in their moments of need. Their mere presence serves as a testament to an unspoken promise–you are seen, you are heard, you matter.

This role, dear friends, goes beyond the confines of traditional religious duties. A chaplain's responsibility is to each patient's unique spiritual tapestry, honoring their beliefs, traditions, and value systems. Whether a person clings to the scriptures of age-old religions, finds solace in the sanctity of nature, or draws strength from a personal creed, the chaplain serves as an affirming and validating companion.

A vital part of a chaplain's work is facilitating spiritual reconciliation. This can involve helping individuals find peace with their life experiences, reaffirming their faith or beliefs, or assisting them in bestowing blessings to their loved ones. Chaplains can also guide family members in offering words of love, forgiveness, or farewell, fostering a sense of closure and peace.

Chaplains are no strangers to the heart's language. They have a unique ability to listen to the unspoken, understanding the subtle nuances of fear, regret, hope, and love. They are trained to recognize and respond to the emotional and spiritual distress that often accompanies terminal illness, providing counsel and comfort to those grappling with questions of life, death, and existence.

However, the role of a chaplain extends far beyond the individual patient. They often serve as a cornerstone for the entire family, offering guidance and support as they traverse the shifting landscapes of anticipatory grief and bereavement. They provide a safe space for expressing emotions, discussing fears, and sharing memories, fostering connections that fortify against the pain of loss.

In the grand tapestry of hospice care, chaplains add the threads of spiritual wellness and existential peace. Their role bridges the gap between medical care and soul care, offering a holistic approach that recognizes the full spectrum of human needs. Steadfast and compassionate, they embody a spirit of gentle resilience, serving as a touchstone of comfort, dignity, and peace in the face of life's most profound transition.

Reflection Questions: Hospice Care Team

1. Identify three key discussions you'd want to have with an RN Case Manager or Doctor for your loved one.

   _____

   _____

   _____

2. List three ways you'd personalize the hospice environment to make your loved one feel at home.

   _____

   _____

   _____

3. Write down three questions you'd ask a Social Worker or Chaplain to ensure they align with your family's needs during this journey.

   _____

   _____

   _____

Caregivers

When it comes to hospice care, it is natural for both patients and caregivers to experience fears and resistance. These emotions often stem from the unknown and the misconceptions surrounding hospice. By shedding light on these common fears, we can work towards dispelling them and creating a more supportive environment for all involved.

Common Fears and Resistance
to Hospice Services

Fear of the Unknown: Facing the end of life can be overwhelming, and entering hospice care can amplify these feelings of uncertainty. Patients and caregivers may fear the loss of control, unfamiliar medical procedures, and the emotional challenges that come with the final stages of life. It is important to address these fears by providing clear and honest information about the hospice process, allowing individuals to better understand what to expect.

Resistance to Letting Go: For some patients and caregivers, accepting the transition to hospice care can be difficult. There may be a sense of resistance to giving up hope or a belief that seeking hospice care means abandoning the fight against the illness. It is crucial to emphasize that hospice care is not about giving up but rather shifting the focus to comfort, quality of life, and dignified end-of-life care.

Fear of Burdening Others: Caregivers often experience a deep sense of responsibility and may worry about burdening their loved ones or healthcare professionals with the demands of caregiving. They may hesitate to seek hospice services because they fear being perceived as incapable or imposing on others. These concerns can be alleviated by educating caregivers about the support available through hospice care, such as respite services and the involvement of trained professionals.

Financial Concerns: The cost of healthcare can be a significant source of anxiety for patients and caregivers. Many may worry about the financial implications of hospice care and the impact it will have on their resources. It is important to address these concerns by providing information about insurance coverage, Medicaid, and Medicare benefits. Assuring individuals that hospice care will be provided even if patients have no payer source. A needy patient will receive the same quality of care as any other patient with a payment source.

Emotional Reservations: Facing the end of life can trigger complex emotions, including grief, fear, and sadness. Patients and caregivers may have reservations about entering hospice care, fearing it will intensify their emotional struggles. By offering emotional support and counseling services as part of hospice care, individuals can find comfort and guidance in navigating these challenging emotions.

Cultural and Religious Beliefs: Cultural and religious beliefs can influence perceptions of hospice care. Some individuals may hold beliefs that conflict with certain aspects of hospice, such as the use of pain medication or end-of-life decision-making. Sensitivity to diverse cultural and religious perspectives is essential, and providing education and open dialogue can help bridge any gaps in understanding.

Perception of Abandonment: Both patients and caregivers may fear that entering hospice care means being left alone or forgotten. They may worry that the support they have received throughout their medical journey will suddenly disappear. It is crucial to emphasize the hospice team's continuous presence, dedication to providing compassionate care, and commitment to ensuring the patient's comfort and well-being until the very end.

By acknowledging these common fears and resistance to hospice services, we can foster an environment of empathy, understanding, and support. Open communication, education, and emotional guidance are integral to addressing these concerns and empowering individuals to embrace the benefits of hospice care.

Existing Roles Stay the Same

Caregivers, whether family, friends, or professional aids, form the unsung chorus in the symphony of hospice care. Their role can be as tender as a whisper, as powerful as a declaration of commitment, bearing witness to a patient's needs, and echoing them to the medical team.

As the caregiver's world synchronizes with the rhythm of hospice care, they may often grapple with uncertainty. These common fears and resistance towards hospice services spring from the unfamiliar and can cast a shadow on the path ahead. But remember, dear caregiver, that hospice services come not to replace but to extend a helping hand to fortify the pre-existing structures of care.

As a patient transitions into hospice care, the caregiver's roles may gain new hues, but the essence remains intact. The acts of feeding, hygiene, and companionship—the melodies of love, compassion, and shared histories—continue to echo within the sanctuary of care. The hospice team becomes an extension, a reinforcement of these loving gestures, amplifying the strength and resilience inherent in every caregiver.

Yet, amidst this critical role, caregivers must observe certain practices that enhance their journey of care. Firstly, remember the patient's wishes are sacred. They are the map guiding you, the melody guiding your dance. Acknowledge, respect, and seek to fulfill them, for they embody the essence of the person you're caring for.

Secondly, understand your own strengths. You, dear caregiver, are a tower of capability, fortified by love and commitment. Doubts may cloud your mind, but beneath it resides a reservoir of resilience, patience, and tenacity. Harness it, for it fuels your capacity to give.

Thirdly, recognize the signposts pointing towards the need for help. It is not a sign of weakness but a testament to your humanity. Reach out to the hospice team, other family members, or support groups. They stand ready to share your load, to offer solace, guidance, and respite.

Finally, be prepared to respond swiftly. The terrain of hospice care is often shifting, and the patient's needs can change in the blink of an eye. Stay alert to their signals, trust your intuition, and liaise with the hospice team to ensure timely intervention.

Navigating the role of a caregiver requires a balance of strength and vulnerability, empathy, and self-care. It is a testament to the depth of human connection and love's unwavering resilience.

Best Practices for Caregivers

I have identified the four best practices for caregivers to acknowledge and follow, as much as possible, when taking care of hospice patients.

1. Understand and honor the wishes of the patient.
2. Understand that you are capable.
3. Know when to ask for help.
4. Be prepared to take quick action.

Honoring the Wishes of the Patient (A True Story / Case Study)

I remember the profound journey of a woman who had birthed not just one or two, but nine children into this world. These children, mostly strong-willed daughters, mirrored her strength and echoed her love for family and life. The woman, having weathered many a storm, had arrived at a juncture where she had to make choices that were both personal and poignant. Her weary yet valiant heart communicated a message that was hard for her to convey: She did not wish to be brought back to life if her heart chose to rest.

And then there was food, once a source of nourishment and joy, now merely a symbol of obligation. Her body no longer desired sustenance in the traditional sense, but her heart wrestled with the worry of disappointing her loved ones. She confided in her hospice nurse, expressing her secret struggle of maintaining appearances at the dining table, taking bites for the sake of others rather than herself. This was a battle she did not wish to fight anymore.

In this intimate dance between personal choice and family dynamics, the role of the hospice social worker proved invaluable. With a heart full of empathy and armed with the wisdom of professional training, the Social Worker held space for the family to navigate these new, uncharted waters. Through patient discussions and gently unfolding revelations, she guided them to see the truth their matriarch was living: The choice to eat or not to eat had to be hers, echoing her inner rhythm rather than the clock on the wall.

The process was akin to peeling back layers of an artichoke, each layer unveiling deeper understanding, acceptance, and eventually, peace. It was not without its challenges, with the family's initial resistance giving way to grudging acceptance and respect for their beloved mother's wishes. In the end, the woman was given the liberty to eat according to her body's desires, not her family's expectations.

The beauty of this narrative lies in its heartening conclusion. Now comfortable in her truth, the patient found a new lease on life, even as it neared its end. And her family, though initially resistant, finally respected her desires. They learned that the most beautiful way to express their love was to honor her decisions, a testament to the boundless capacity of human understanding and love.

Understand that You Are Capable (A True Story / Case Study)

I recollect the tale of a son's unwavering devotion to his mother, his dedication encapsulating the boundless power of love. A gentleman once reached out to our services, his voice reflecting a palpable anxiety. He queried about the availability of our Certified Nursing Assistants over the weekend, the very weekend we typically reserve for patients on our Sacred Journey Care Program or those nearing the twilight of their lives.

His story was simple yet profound; his mother had fallen, and he had painstakingly hoisted her frail body back onto the bed, cleansing her with care. Still, a worry lingered in his heart, an unsettling fear that his efforts might have been insufficient. Even though his concerns didn't meet the standard criteria for an emergency, his voice echoed a plea that touched my heart. Without a promise but with a silent determination, I decided to check on his mother. I reasoned that if a true crisis unfolded elsewhere, my route would need to change.

Upon reaching their home, I was met with his warm greeting. I noticed beads of sweat adorning his forehead, painting a picture of an arduous struggle behind closed doors. I braced myself for the sight that awaited me, a picture of disarray and discomfort. But what unfolded was an extraordinary testimony to love, care, and resilience.

The gentleman had painstakingly restored order amidst the initial chaos. He had replaced his mother's soiled clothes, scrubbed the scene of the fall to its former neatness, and bathed his mother till she sparkled. He went a step further, dusting her chest with comforting powder, a touch as tender as a mother's caress. The sight of this elderly lady, impeccably clean and comfortably ensconced in her bed, touched the depths of my heart.

The raw emotions threatened to break free, a surge of respect and awe threatening to spill as tears. This man, the only child of a single mother, reciprocated her love and care in a manner both admirable and heartwarming. His meticulous attention to her needs, his gentle demeanor, and his ability to step up when duty called was a testament to his capability and strength. It served as a reminder that we often possess more strength than we realize and that we are indeed capable, even when faced with overwhelming circumstances.

Know When to Ask for Help
(A True Story / Case Study)

I share the story of Jennifer, a testament to the necessity of seeking assistance when the weight of responsibility becomes overbearing. Jennifer, an only child now immersed in her own family life, made the compassionate choice to bring her ailing mother under her roof. She yearned to shield her mother from the sterile and impersonal environment of a hospital in her twilight days. However, the ripples of her decision soon began to touch every corner of her existence.

Weeks cascaded into one another, each bringing the harsh realization that her mother's care was casting an increasingly heavy toll on her family's equilibrium and her own mental sanctity. Yet, Jennifer remained steadfast, resolute in her decision to keep her mother within the comforting confines of home. Her life became a tableau of tireless devotion, her entire being consumed by the act of caring.

Hospice care offers a respite service, a lifeline for caregivers teetering on the edge of exhaustion. It promises a temporary sanctuary for patients, allowing caregivers to retreat and rejuvenate for five consecutive days. Jennifer was acutely aware of this offering, yet the fortitude of her spirit wavered, pushing her towards a precipice she hadn't foreseen. She found herself in the throes of a mental breakdown, the weariness of her soul rendering her incapable of continuing her caregiving journey.

During this crisis, the hospice social worker stepped in, an embodiment of the assistance that Jennifer had been reluctant to seek. The social worker orchestrated respite care for the patient, providing Jennifer with the desperately needed breathing space. This solution was a temporary balm, a bridge leading toward the eventual availability of a nursing home placement.

Jennifer's tale underscores the imperative of recognizing when we need to extend our hands for help. It speaks volumes about the strength embedded in the act of seeking assistance. As caregivers, it is crucial to remember that our ability to care for others often hinges on our own well-being. Thus, knowing when to pause and ask for help is an act of self-preservation and, ultimately, a testament to our love for those we care for.

Taking Quick Action
(A True Story / Case Study)

It was the wee hours of the morning, around two a.m., when my phone buzzed to life with a call from a distressed caregiver. Her mother was wrestling with relentless seizures, a storm of convulsions that had held her captive throughout the night. The caregiver, her daughter, reached out with urgency, seeking guidance on how to navigate this turbulent chapter.

Having been the primary caregiver, she had already demonstrated admirable responsiveness by administering the prescribed anti-seizure medications orally. Yet, the escalating severity of the situation had thrust a formidable barrier in their path—her mother was no longer able to swallow the medication. A seemingly insurmountable challenge loomed before them.

The conversation took an unexpected turn when the on-call nurse suggested an alternate method of medication administration: rectally. To this, the caregiver bravely consented without a moment's hesitation. With the guiding voice of the nurse echoing in her ear, she traversed unfamiliar terrain and swiftly administered the much-needed medication.

The ripple effects of her immediate intervention were profoundly palpable. By the time the hospice nurse visited later that morning, the patient was comfortably nestled within the familiar confines of her home. The seizing storm had subsided, and her symptoms managed effectively to prevent further escalation. The sight that greeted the nurse was one of serene tranquility, a far cry from the turbulent scenario painted over the phone just hours ago. The caregiver's prompt action effectively averted a crisis, ensuring that her mother did not have to endure prolonged suffering while waiting for professional medical help.

This narrative illuminates how the daughter courageously stepped into an unfamiliar role and surpassed her own expectations. The enormity of her capacity for care was evident in her ability to endure, adapt, and overcome, manifesting an extraordinary blend of courage, adaptability, and resilience. The end result? Her mother didn't need to be rushed to the hospital; she could rest in the comfort of her home as she desired. She remained at peace, her comfort protected by her daughter's swift, decisive action.

In hospice care, such instances emphasize the power of immediate action. Often, it is this preparedness and presence of mind that spells the difference between discomfort and relief, between fear and reassurance, and ultimately, between life and death. To caregivers everywhere, let this be a potent reminder of your innate capacity and the significant impact of your immediate action.

Common Caregiver Abuses

It is vital to emphasize that caregiver abuses, while not commonplace, do occur and need to be openly acknowledged and appropriately addressed. Often, the manifestations of these abuses arise from varying circumstances, such as an inability to effectively juggle caregiving duties with other responsibilities, lack of financial savviness, or the emotional and mental strain associated with caregiving. In certain extreme situations, it may stem from a lack of regard for the patient's well-being or vested self-interests.

Neglecting Patients:
The Struggle between Care and Responsibilities
Life is a balancing act, a reality that particularly rings true for caregivers. In the beginning, the act of caregiving tends to be less demanding. Patients are often more capable of managing themselves with only part-time assistance. However, the patient's needs escalate as the disease advances, requiring more intense care. Eventually, in the hospice stage, round-the-clock care becomes essential.

Sadly, caregivers often find themselves unable to provide this level of commitment due to other obligations, primarily work. It's not an uncommon sight for social workers to come across patients left alone without adequate care. Reactions to this reality can range from denial and defensiveness to guilt-ridden acceptance.

Consider the case of Helen, a single mother balancing a demanding job and her duty as a caregiver to her ailing father. Helen would leave her father alone during work hours, hoping he'd manage himself. It took intervention from a social worker for Helen to realize the severity of her actions and the potential risk to her father. Following discussions, Helen was able to arrange for a neighbor to check in on her father during her work hours, providing him with the required attention.

Misappropriation of Funds:
Financial Exploitation

Financial abuses within the realm of caregiving are unfortunately prevalent and take on different forms. From using the patient's money for personal indulgence or paying off debts to supporting addictive habits and unscrupulous loans, these abuses reflect a lack of financial literacy and an absence of moral integrity.

One stark example is of a patient named George, whose nephew had assumed the role of caregiver. With time, the nephew started to misuse George's funds for his own purposes, paying off personal debts and even funding a lavish vacation. Only after an intervention by a vigilant social worker did the situation come to light, leading to the nephew's removal from his caregiving role.

Physical Abuse and Beyond: The Dark Side of Caregiving

Physical abuse, while less common, can be a manifestation of accumulated frustration, resentment, or underlying mental health issues. But abuse extends beyond the physical. The emotional, psychological, and verbal mistreatment of patients is a grim reality.

A distressing incident involved a terminally ill hospice patient, Mary, who died after mysteriously falling down the stairs. An investigation revealed that her husband, her primary caregiver, had pushed her. His motives were unclear, but the tragic incident remains a harsh reminder of the potential dangers that caregivers with malevolent intentions pose.

Upholding the Sanctity of the Caregiving Role

Working in the death industry requires individuals to maintain a positive outlook despite the difficult circumstances. Encountering instances of abuse or cold-heartedness can challenge this perspective. In these situations, it becomes crucial to remember the compassionate, empathetic caregivers who fulfill their roles with grace and dedication.

It is essential to address caregiver abuse firmly and promptly to ensure the safety and well-being of the patients under their care. Each case serves as a stark reminder of the importance of proper support, education, and monitoring in the caregiving process to prevent these abuses and uphold the sanctity of the caregiving role.

Reflection Questions: Caregivers

1. Which aspect of hospice care feels most unfamiliar or daunting to you?

_____

_____

_____

2. Is there a particular hospice myth or misconception that's been lingering in your mind? Write it out.

_____

_____

_____

3. Have you had any previous experiences with hospice? If so, what emotions or memories arise?

_____

_____

_____

Common Hospice Myths

There's a palpable sense of unease that enshrouds the very term "hospice care." It's tinged with misconceptions and inaccuracies that form a thick fog, obscuring the true essence of this vital service. It's tragic because these misconceptions, these damaging myths, deprive those in need of the grace, peace, and dignity that hospice care can bring during life's final chapter.

Each of us must challenge the myths and deconstruct them piece by piece to bring clarity and understanding. The reality of hospice care is beautiful in its raw sincerity. It's about preserving the dignity of life even as it ebbs away and offering a haven of tranquility amidst the tempest of emotional turmoil. We must shine a piercing light on the truth and drive away the shroud of misunderstanding.

But how? Through conversations grounded in compassion and facts. Our task is to stir dialogues that infuse empathy into the hard truths. We must educate and advocate, for it is through awareness that transformation truly begins. When we open up to discussions about the last chapters of life, we can truly appreciate and grasp the essence of hospice care.

There's a particular strength in confronting our fears and misconceptions head-on. But with hospice care, it's not only about strength but also about grace, comfort, and above all else, respect for the journey of life that every individual is on. Misconceptions confuse and can turn into fear. Fear, in turn, pushes us to avoid these conversations. But avoidance doesn't lead us anywhere. It's like treading water in a vast sea; you're not moving forward. You're just exhausting yourself.

So, let's be the change. Let's lift the veil off hospice care. Let's dispel the myths and embrace the truth. Let's be the lanterns that shine a light on the true essence of hospice care. Let's normalize the conversations, infuse them with compassion, and bring clarity to those who need it the most.

We stand on the precipice of a new understanding, a new acceptance. Every myth we debunk, every truth we shine a light on, and every conversation we have brings us a step closer to the heart of what hospice care truly is—a beacon of peace, comfort, and dignity during life's most profound transition. It's time for us to courageously step forward and embrace the truth about hospice care. Let's dive in together.

The Misconception That Hospice is a Place

One of the most widespread misconceptions about hospice care is the notion that hospice is a physical location. A place, much like a hospital or a nursing home, where patients are taken to spend their final days. However, the reality is quite different. Hospice is a form of service, a system of specialized care, that is rendered wherever the patient calls home. This could be in the patient's own house, a nursing facility, or an assisted living residence.

Often, families feel overwhelmed when their loved ones require constant care. In their search for help, they come across the term "hospice" and start to think about it as a destination, somewhere they could move their loved one to, hoping that there, the much-needed care will be provided. However, this is simply not the case.

To illustrate, imagine a patient, we'll call him Jim, who has been battling cancer for years. When the disease progresses to a point where curative treatment is no longer effective, Jim's doctor might suggest hospice care. But this doesn't mean that Jim would be relocated to a "hospice." Instead, a hospice care team would start providing services at Jim's current residence, bringing to him all the necessary medical, spiritual, and emotional support.

The Misunderstanding Around Morphine Usage

The use of morphine in hospice care is another area that is often misunderstood. Morphine, a powerful pain reliever, is commonly used in hospice care to alleviate severe pain and breathing difficulties. However, there are two widespread myths related to morphine use that need to be dispelled.

Myth:
Hospice Can Administer Lethal Doses of Morphine

Some people believe that hospice care providers can administer any amount of morphine, even if it's a lethal dose, to hasten a patient's death. However, this is far from the truth. Hospice care is a highly regulated field, and providers are not permitted to administer lethal doses of any medications.

Hospice aims not to hasten death but to provide comfort, alleviate suffering, and enhance the quality of life in a patient's remaining days. Comparing the process of dying to childbirth may provide a better understanding of this. During childbirth, an epidural might be administered for pain relief. Regardless of whether the mother receives an epidural or not, the baby is coming. In the same way, death is inevitable for a person in the final stages of life.

The use of medications like morphine in hospice care (akin to the epidural) is meant to help the patient experience this process with minimal discomfort.

Myth:

Morphine Causes Premature Death

Another misbelief that people hold is that the administration of morphine leads to premature death. As a patient's health declines and they are nearing their final stages, morphine is often administered to provide comfort during the process. The timing of these doses may create a misconception. In many cases, morphine is administered shortly before a patient's death, but this is because experienced hospice nurses, who are in tune with the stages of dying, anticipate worsening symptoms and administer the drug accordingly.

The correlation between morphine administration and symptom escalation is often misunderstood. The truth is that as symptoms worsen due to the natural progression of the disease, more morphine may be needed to manage the discomfort. However, the morphine is not causing the symptoms to worsen; it's simply responding to the worsening symptoms.

The Caregivers' Role Continues Unchanged

When a patient enters hospice care, one of the common misconceptions is that the caregiver's role ends. However, this is far from the truth. Whether the caregiver is a family member, friend, or professional nursing staff, their role continues even after the patient has entered hospice care.

The main duties of a hospice team include managing the patient's pain and symptoms, providing emotional and spiritual support, offering therapies like physiotherapy or occupational therapy as needed, and delivering necessary medical supplies and equipment. However, caregivers continue to play a significant role in providing daily personal care, like bathing, feeding, grooming, and emotional support.

The Misconception About IV Nutrition

As patients near the end of their lives, their bodies gradually start to shut down. One sign of this process is a decrease in appetite or even a complete lack of interest in food. However, caregivers often misinterpret this and believe that the patient needs to be given nutrition intravenously (IV). This myth, albeit coming from a place of concern and care, can inadvertently lead to more harm than good.

The reality is that as the body shuts down, it no longer requires the same amount of nutrition as it once did. By forcing nutrition through an IV, it can cause excess fluid to build up in the body, particularly in the lungs, leading to difficulty in breathing—a condition referred to as a "wet death." On the other hand, patients who are allowed to pass without the burden of excess fluids or nutrition are said to experience a 'dry death', which is often less distressing.

The Importance of Preventative Approach to Pain Management

It's not uncommon for caregivers and patients to think that pain medications should only be administered when pain is present. However, a preventative approach to pain management often proves to be most effective when it comes to end-of-life care.

As pain intensifies, it becomes harder to control. So, when pain is anticipated, preemptive use of medication can help keep the pain at bay.

Myth:
All hospices provide the same service

Hospices are not created equal. Although the philosophy of hospice is to provide care and compassion for those facing a life-limiting illness, the specific services offered by each hospice may vary.

In choosing a hospice, caregivers should do their due diligence to identify the services offered, the hospice's reputation, and how well they meet the patient's specific needs.

For instance, some hospices may provide complementary therapies such as massage, art, pet, and music therapy. Others may have spiritual counselors on staff to meet the spiritual needs of patients and their families. The staffing ratios, such as the number of patients per nurse or social worker, may also vary among hospices.

Selecting a hospice is a very personal choice. There is no one-size-fits-all solution. The key is to find a hospice that fits the patient's needs and values and that will provide the level of care required to ensure their comfort and dignity during the end of life.

Hospice is a service focused on patient comfort and improving quality of life during the end-of-life journey. The myths and misconceptions about hospice care may prevent people from accessing this crucial service. By debunking these myths and sharing the truth about hospice, we can help more people benefit from hospice's compassionate, patient-centered care. To truly appreciate the beauty of a sunset, one must face west.

Final Thoughts

Together, we have navigated through the unspoken, the misunderstood, and the often-feared journey of hospice care. We've found that beneath the layers of discomfort, anxiety, and doubt, there lies a reservoir of strength, compassion, and profound understanding. It is my sincere hope that this work served not just as a guide but as a beacon of hope.

The echoes of this journey reverberate in each word, each phrase, and each lesson contained within these pages. The knowledge acquired here is not merely about symptom management, though that is a critical component. No, it goes deeper than that. It is about infusing vibrancy into each day, each moment, even as we are faced with the reality of life's fragility. It's about understanding that while we may not be able to add more days to life, we can add more life to each day for both patients and caregivers.

To our brave caregivers, the silent heroes in the backdrop, this book is a testament to your strength, your resilience, and your unwavering compassion. It is a reflection of your determination to stand as a pillar of strength, providing comfort, support, and love to those entrusted in your care. From the knowledge gleaned on avoiding burnout to the understanding of the wealth of respite services at your disposal, this book was designed to equip you for the road ahead, as arduous as it may sometimes be.

To the patients embarking on this journey, I hope this book serves as your compass, guiding you through the myriad of questions, fears, and uncertainties that often accompany this stage of life. From understanding your symptoms to reaching out for the help you need, I expect this book will continue to provide the clarity you need even amidst the chaos.

But our journey in this book doesn't end with patients and caregivers. It extends to nurses, administrators, and the entire ecosystem that forms the backbone of hospice care. Use this book as a resource, a repository of knowledge and wisdom to enhance the compassionate care you provide to your patients.

While the chapters of this book may have come to an end, the journey continues. The lessons learned, the insights gleaned, and the wisdom imparted continue to guide us on our paths. This book, while a finite collection of pages, is but a snapshot of a larger narrative—one of resilience, compassion, strength, and the profound humanity that lies at the heart of hospice care.

As you step away from this shared experience, remember that the echoes of this journey linger long after the last word is read. The wisdom embedded within these pages transcends beyond the realm of hospice care and seeps into the fabric of our lives, reminding us to live fully, love deeply, and appreciate each moment, each breath, and each heartbeat.

As the curtain falls on this chapter, remember that in the grand symphony of life, your melody matters. Your strength, your compassion, your resilience, and your humanity are the notes that enrich the harmonious score of life. Keep these lessons close to your heart, and allow them to guide, inspire, and enlighten you. And as you traverse through your sacred journey, remember to be present, be compassionate, be patient, and above all, be kind to yourself. Your journey, though marked with challenges, is beautiful in its own unique way. Embrace it, cherish it, and find comfort in knowing that you are not alone on this path. You are seen. You are valued. You are loved.

Petergay

Reflection Questions: Common Hospice Myths

1. Reflect on one hospice myth you believed before reading this chapter. How has your perspective changed? Take a moment to jot down your insights.

   _____

   _____

   _____

2. Consider any hesitations or fears you may have had about hospice care. Which myths fueled these feelings? Outline three ways to address these concerns in future discussions.

   _____

   _____

   _____

3. How would you handle a situation where a loved one believes a hospice myth? List two steps.

   _____

   _____

   _____

Sacred Journey Consulting

Services for Individuals and Families

Not everyone who searches for information on hospice care is immediately embarking on that journey. Some are simply researching ahead, seeking information in the face of a life-limiting illness, or exploring options for loved ones. The internet is a wealth of information, but it can also be overwhelming. This is where my consultation comes in.

My role as a consultant isn't only to provide information but to clarify, simplify, and personalize it. I help individuals decode the complexity of hospice care, provide clear answers, and shed light on the nuances that generic information often misses. By guiding individuals through this labyrinth of information, they gain the knowledge they need to make informed decisions about hospice care.

Understanding Hospice Care

Hospice care is more than medical care; it's a comprehensive approach that considers the physical, emotional, social, and spiritual needs of patients. It's about living as well as possible for as long as possible, providing comfort and dignity in the face of a life-limiting illness. But many don't understand this.

Part of my service involves dispelling the myths around hospice care. It's not about giving up or waiting to die but embracing a new phase of life and making the most out of it. By redefining hospice care, individuals can see it as a source of support and care, rather than a sign of defeat.

Navigating the System

Another crucial aspect of my consultation service for information seekers is helping them navigate the system. The hospice care system can be daunting with its myriad of services, regulations, and processes. It's easy to feel lost and overwhelmed.

In my consultation, I simplify the complexities of the system, making it more accessible and easier to understand. I guide individuals through the eligibility criteria, the admission process, care plans, and what to expect during the journey. More importantly, I empower them with the tools and knowledge to advocate for their needs or the needs of their loved ones within the system.

Evaluating Care Providers

Selecting a hospice care provider is a crucial decision. However, not all providers are created equal. Different hospices offer different services, have different approaches, and achieve different outcomes. But how can one make an informed choice?

My consultation service can assist in this crucial step. Based on years of experience in the field, I provide guidance on evaluating hospice care providers, understanding their service offerings, and comparing their strengths and weaknesses. I assist individuals in identifying the right fit for their needs or the needs of their loved ones.

Transitioning to Hospice Care

Transitioning to hospice care is often an emotionally charged time. The decision comes with a mix of emotions—relief, acceptance, fear, sadness, and sometimes guilt. It's a time when support and guidance can make a big difference.

As a consultant, I offer a compassionate, empathetic ear and a calming voice amidst the turmoil. I provide emotional support, assist in managing the transition, and offer guidance on coping strategies for both patients and their families.

My services at Sacred Journey Consulting are designed to enlighten, empower, and guide individuals and organizations in their hospice journey. Whether it's corporate decision-makers striving to improve their services, case managers working tirelessly to deliver care, patients and families navigating this new phase of life, or individuals seeking clarity amidst a sea of information, I am here to serve, guide, and walk this sacred journey with you. Your journey matters, and together, we can make it a journey of peace, dignity, and quality living.

Services for Corporate Decision-Makers in Hospice Organizations

Strategic Advising and Consultation

Hospice care is an intricate sector with its own unique challenges and opportunities. Navigating this sector successfully demands a comprehensive understanding of the dynamics involved and the ability to make strategic decisions based on that understanding. My role as a strategic advisor is to equip you with the information, insights, and tools you need to make informed, effective decisions that steer your organization toward success.

Operational Optimization

Efficiency and effectiveness are paramount in hospice care. Every wasted resource or missed opportunity can impact the quality of care provided. My services include a thorough assessment of your operations, identifying areas of improvement, and developing strategies to optimize your resources. I can help streamline processes, improve team communication, and foster a culture of continuous improvement, enhancing both the productivity of your team and the quality of care provided.

Staff Development and Training

Your team is your most valuable asset, and investing in their development is vital. I offer tailored training programs to equip your staff with the skills and knowledge needed to deliver exceptional hospice care. These programs cover a broad spectrum of topics, including patient care techniques, emotional resilience, self-care, and team collaboration.

Moreover, I also provide guidance on staff retention strategies, creating a supportive work environment, and fostering a culture of empathy and compassion.

Policy and Compliance Guidance

Navigating the legal and regulatory landscape of hospice care can be complex. Compliance with relevant laws and regulations is essential to avoid legal consequences and maintain the trust of patients and families. My services include guidance on policy development and adherence to regulatory standards, ensuring your organization remains compliant while providing the best possible care.

Strategic Partnerships and Networking

Building strategic partnerships is vital in hospice care. Whether it's partnering with other healthcare providers, community organizations, or policymakers, such partnerships can greatly enhance your hospice's reach and impact. I can help you identify potential partnership opportunities, negotiate agreements, and build fruitful, long-lasting relationships in the hospice care sector.

My goal with these services is not just to improve the operational aspects of your hospice organization but to create a nurturing environment where compassionate care can flourish. By working together, we can ensure your hospice organization is well-equipped to provide high-quality, compassionate care to those at the end of their life's journey.

About the Author

Petergay Dunkley-Mullings has demonstrated success as a hospice nurse and manager, as a parent, as a wife, as an immigrant, and as a non-profit leader. She has a strong track record of success and is a role model to many.

With a desire to leverage her experience in hospice care, she has prepared Hospice Sense to guide patients, caregivers, and families through this final journey. Hospice is a passion of Petergay's. She loves taking care of patients, and their families and friends, through their end-of-life transition.

As a self-described workaholic, Petergay has worked two jobs for as long as she can remember. Additionally, Petergay operates a non-profit organization. The foundation currently supports twenty-two students from eleven parishes, and Petergay works tirelessly to ensure these young adults can stay in school. Each student has a sponsor and a mentor who guides them to achieving their specific goal.

You can learn more about Petergay in her memoir, Can't Afford to Fail. She is a TEDx speaker, a transformational coach, and the recipient of The Jamaica Beacon Award 2023. She also appeared on the Atlanta CW-69, CVM-TV, multiple radio programs, magazines, and podcasts.

She desires to deliver the hospice message to the world because everyone will have to deal with some type of end-of-life decision. As an expert in the field, she offers valuable tips to hospice organizations, as well as individuals, to help the dying live their last days as their best days.

Notes

Notes

Notes

Notes

_____

_____

_____

_____

_____

_____

_____

_____

_____

_____

_____

_____

_____

_____

_____

_____

_____

_____

Notes

Notes

Made in United States
Orlando, FL
05 October 2023

37578294R00068